THE
BREAKUP HAIR HANDBOOK

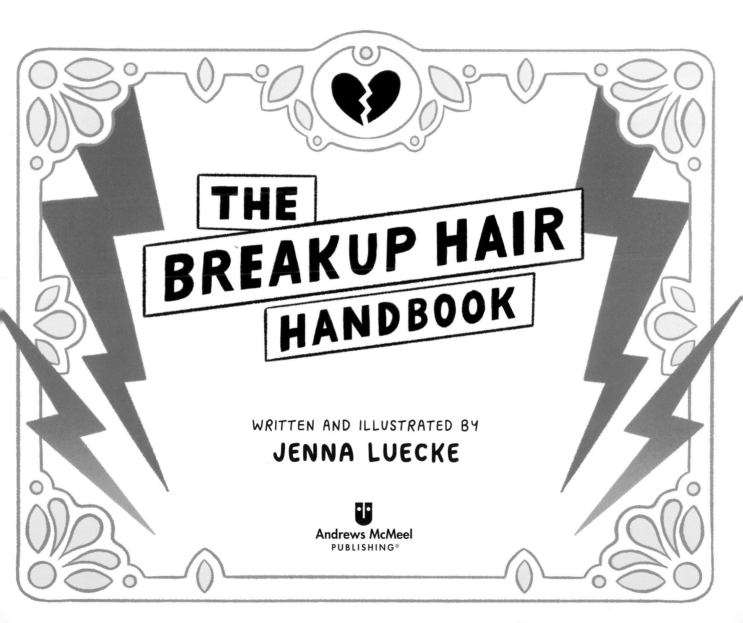

THE BREAKUP HAIR HANDBOOK

WRITTEN AND ILLUSTRATED BY
JENNA LUECKE

Andrews McMeel
PUBLISHING®

TABLE OF CONTENTS

CHOOSING THE CUT

CHOOSING THE COLOR

SO YOU'RE GOING THROUGH A BREAKUP.

AND IT FUCKING SUCKS.

IT WILL PROBABLY MAKE YOU WANT TO DO
ALL KINDS OF CRAZY THINGS, LIKE ADOPT
SEVEN DOGS, BECOME A YOGA INSTRUCTOR,
SELL EVERYTHING YOU OWN, AND LIVE OUT
OF A RENOVATED BUS,

AND, OH YEAH, CHANGE YOUR HAIR.

NOW STOP RIGHT THERE.
LISTEN TO REASON FOR A SECOND.

GIRL, YOU NEED TO . . .

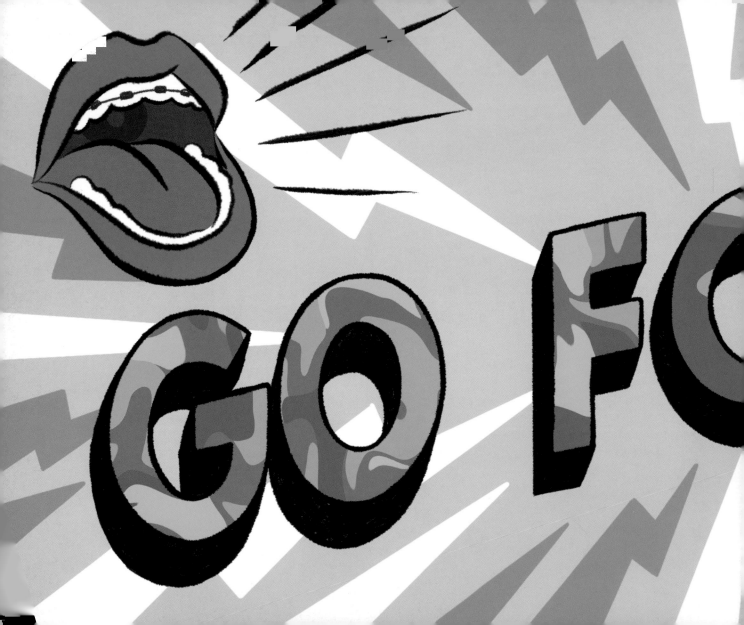

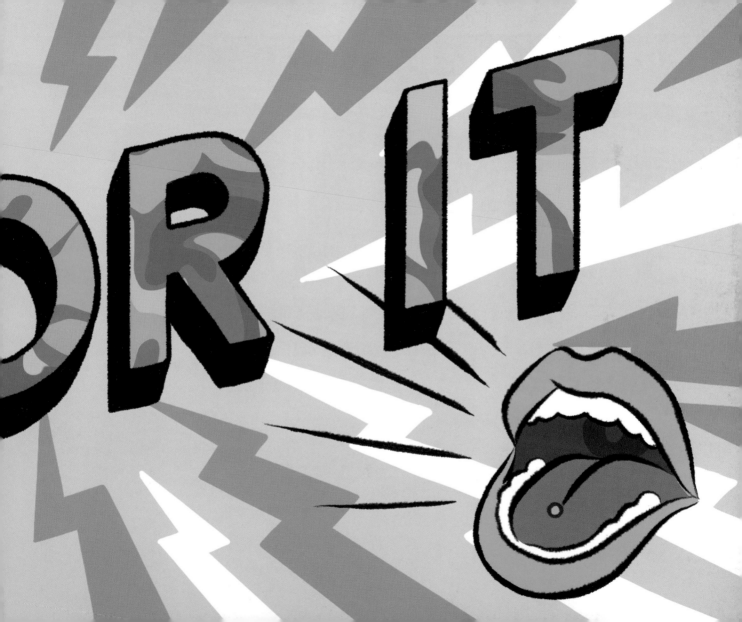

SO HERE'S THE THING.

AS WOMEN, WHEN WE WANT TO CHANGE
OUR HAIR, WE'RE TOLD TO STOP AND THINK
THROUGH EVERY POSSIBLE CONSEQUENCE.
WHETHER OR NOT IT SUITS OUR FACE SHAPE,
WHOM IT MIGHT DISPLEASE, AND WHAT IF
THAT EXTRA THREE MINUTES IT TAKES TO
STRAIGHTEN BANGS *UTTERLY DESTROYS
OUR DAILY ROUTINE AND EVENTUALLY RUINS
OUR LIVES*, ETC.

TOO OFTEN WE ARE LED TO MAKE STYLE CHOICES, ESPECIALLY HAIR CHOICES, OUT OF FEAR. FEAR THAT WE WON'T LOOK ATTRACTIVE ENOUGH, PROFESSIONAL ENOUGH, YOUNG OR OLD ENOUGH, FEMININE ENOUGH. FEAR THAT IT WILL LOOK LIKE WE'RE PUTTING IN TOO MUCH EFFORT OR NOT ENOUGH. **WE'RE TOLD WE NEED TO MOLD OURSELVES TO SOMEONE ELSE'S PREFERENCES, WHETHER IT BE ONE SPECIFIC SOMEONE OR THE WHOLE DAMN WORLD.**

OF COURSE, YOU KNOW THIS ALREADY—YOU
LIVE WITH THESE PRESSURES EVERY DAY.
YOU MIGHT HAVE EVEN ACCEPTED THAT
THIS IS JUST THE WAY IT IS AND YOU HAVE
TO PLAY ALONG. BUT THAT'S WHY RIGHT
NOW IS SUCH A SPECIAL TIME. YOU JUST
HAD YOUR HEART BROKEN, AND YOU'RE DONE
WITH THE BULLSHIT. RIGHT NOW YOU ARE
OUT TO IMPRESS NO ONE, PLEASE NO ONE,
PROVE YOUR WORTH TO NO ONE ... EXCEPT
YOURSELF.

SO GET THE HAIRCUT YOU WANT. DRESS THE WAY YOU WANT. WEAR AS MUCH OR AS LITTLE MAKEUP AS YOU DAMN WELL PLEASE. IF FOR NO OTHER REASON THAN TO REMIND YOURSELF THAT YOU DO NOT BELONG TO ANYONE ELSE—

YOU BELONG TO YOU.

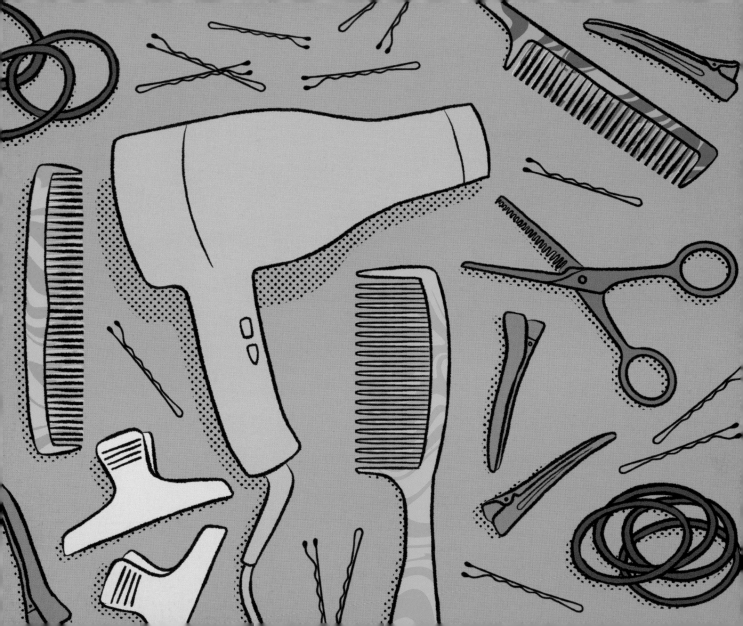

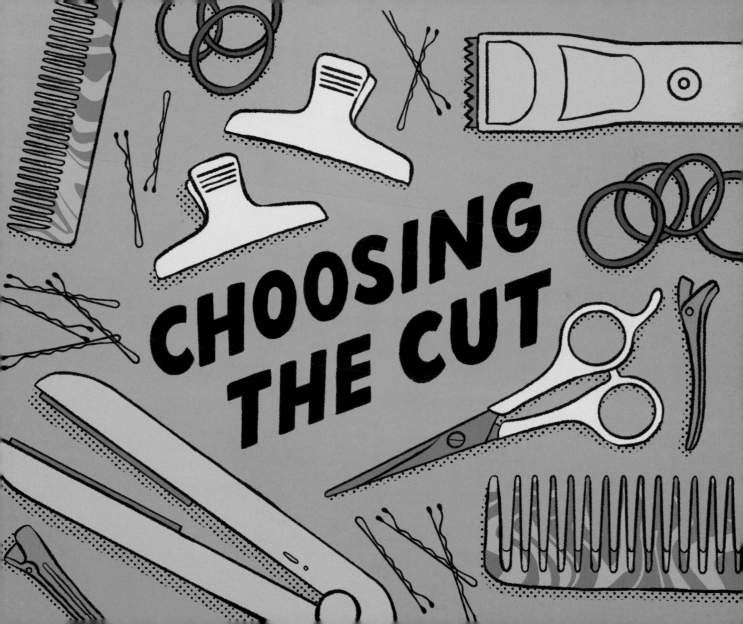

CHOOSING THE CUT

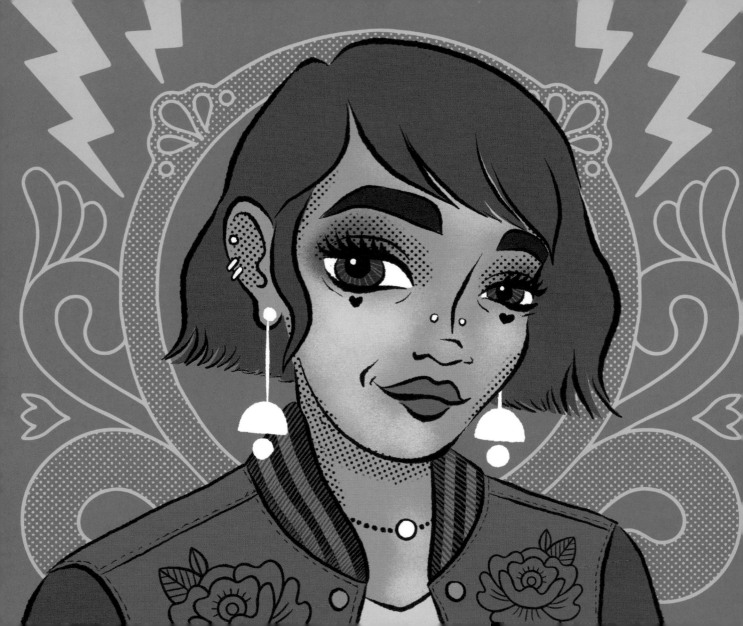

LONG GONE

BOBS AND SHOULDER LENGTH

LONG HAIR MIGHT BE SOCIETY'S IDEAL, BUT IT'S NO LONGER IDEAL FOR YOU. DESPITE THE CONSTANT CROONING THAT YOU HAVE JUST *THE BEST* HAIR, YOU'VE (SECRETLY) BEEN WANTING TO CHOP IT OFF FOR AGES. WHETHER YOU'VE STUCK WITH LONG HAIR BECAUSE YOUR EX PREFERRED IT, BECAUSE YOUR MOTHER INSISTED IT WAS YOUR BEST LOOK, OR BECAUSE EVERY MOVIE YOU'VE SEEN SINCE INFANCY HAS NOT-SO-SUBTLY ASSERTED THAT YOU CANNOT BE THE LEADING LADY WITHOUT WAIST-LENGTH BEACHY WAVES, NONE OF THAT IS ON YOUR MIND NOW. **IT'S TIME TO DITCH THAT LENGTH AND ALL THE BAGGAGE THAT COMES WITH IT.**

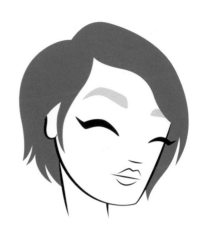

CLASSIC BOB

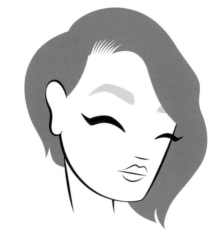

ASYMMETRICAL BOB

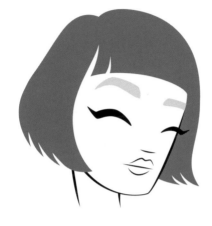

RETRO BOB

REFERENCE PHOTOS

ONCE YOU HAVE A STYLE IN MIND, SCOUR THE INTERNET FOR AS MANY PHOTOS AS YOU NEED TO GET THE IDEA ACROSS TO YOUR STYLIST. "ANGLED BOB" CAN MEAN MANY THINGS TO MANY PEOPLE.

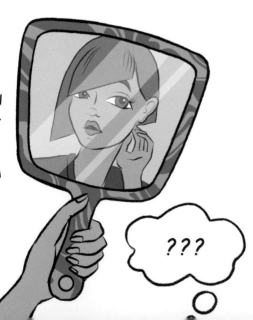

???

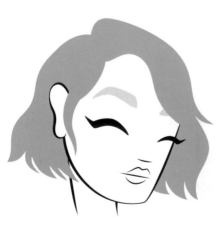

BLUNT CUT

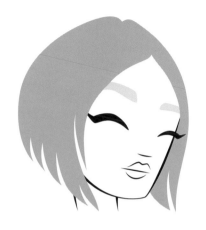

ANGLED BOB

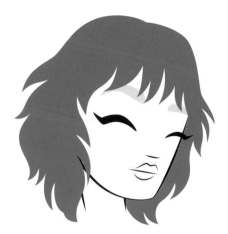

SHAG CUT

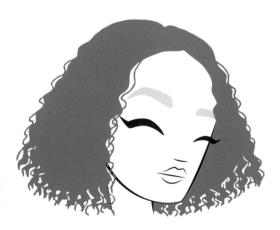

TRIANGLE BOB

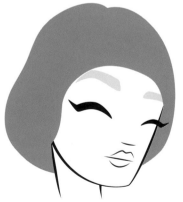

PAGEBOY

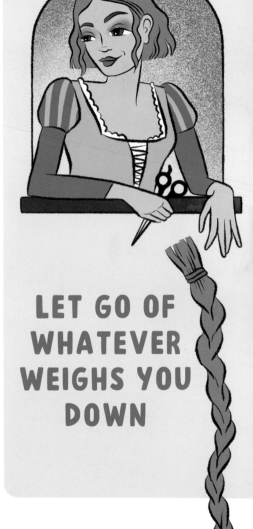

LET GO OF WHATEVER WEIGHS YOU DOWN

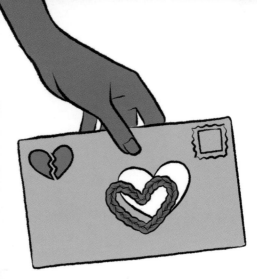

HAIR DONATION

TAKE THOSE LIBERATED LOCKS AND GIVE THEM TO A GOOD CAUSE! NOT ONLY WILL IT MAKE YOU FEEL EVEN BETTER ABOUT YOUR DECISION, IT'S ALSO A GREAT SCAPEGOAT FOR ANYONE GIVING YOU GRIEF FOR CUTTING YOUR LONG HAIR. AUNT LYNDA, *IT WAS FOR CHARITY.*

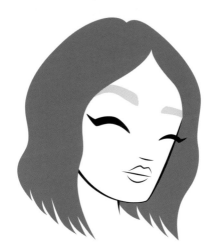

LOB (LONG BOB)

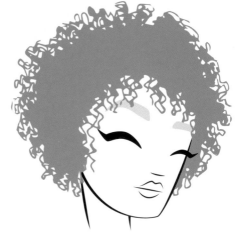

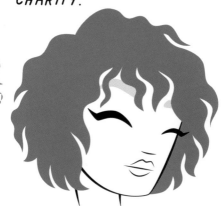

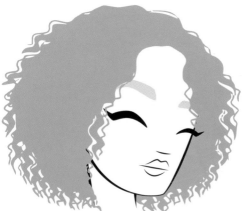

← CURLY BOBS →

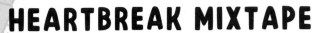

HEARTBREAK MIXTAPE

YOU'RE GOING TO CRY. A LOT. AND INSTEAD OF BOTTLING IT UP UNTIL IT COMES OUT IN, SAY, A MEETING WITH YOUR BOSS, YOU MIGHT AS WELL GET YOUR SOB FESTS OUT WHEN YOU HAVE TIME TO REALLY WALLOW IN THEM. FIND THE "HURTS SO GOOD" SONGS THAT WORK FOR YOU, PUT THAT SHIT ON REPEAT, AND LET IT ALL OUT.

SIDE A: FOR YELLING

PROBABLY IN YOUR CAR WHILE GOING NINETY ON THE HIGHWAY

SINCE U BEEN GONE ● *KELLY CLARKSON*

BAD BLOOD ● *TAYLOR SWIFT*

GIVES YOU HELL ● *THE ALL-AMERICAN REJECTS*

GOOD AS HELL ● *LIZZO*

IRREPLACEABLE ● *BEYONCÉ*

SIDE B: FOR CRYING

PROBABLY IN THE FETAL POSITION ON YOUR BEDROOM FLOOR

THE NIGHT WE MET ● *LORD HURON*

WATCH ME FALL APART ● *SARAH JAFFE*

LANDFILL ● *DAUGHTER*

MAPS ● *YEAH YEAH YEAHS*

BASICALLY ANYTHING BY *THE NATIONAL*

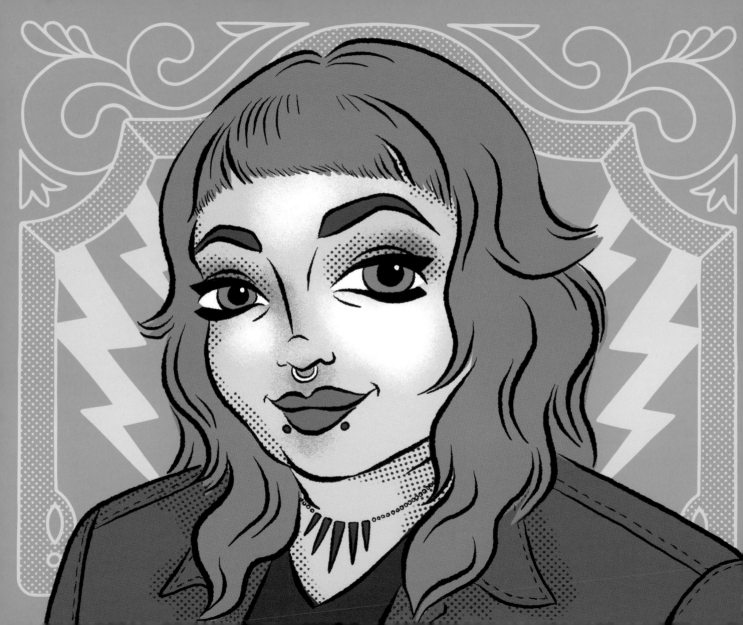

TRIAL SEPARATION

BANGS

BANGS HAVE ALWAYS BEEN SEEN AS THE CLASSIC "PANIC MODE" HAIRCUT. THE HELLO-WORLD-I'M-GOING-THROUGH-A-THING HAIRCUT. AND SO WHAT IF YOU ARE? BANGS ARE EASY TO DO AT HOME AND, YES, SPUR OF THE MOMENT IF THAT'S YOUR VIBE. THEY CAN BE ADDED TO ALMOST ANY STYLE AND MIRACULOUSLY TRANSFORM IT INTO A BRAND-NEW LOOK. WE'RE TALKING "I DIDN'T EVEN RECOGNIZE YOU!"-LEVEL TRANSFORMATION. SO LET'S CLARIFY THIS HERE AND NOW, FOR OURSELVES AND FOR THE WORLD: WOMEN DO NOT GET BANGS AS A CRY FOR HELP—WE GET BANGS BECAUSE **BANGS ARE THE MAGIC FAIRY DUST OF THE HAIRSTYLE REALM**. SO WHETHER YOUR NEW BANGS COME BY WAY OF A SALON APPOINTMENT OR WINE AND A YOUTUBE TUTORIAL AT 1 A.M.: OWN IT, ROCK IT, AND DON'T FEEL THE NEED TO EXPLAIN YOURSELF TO ANYONE.

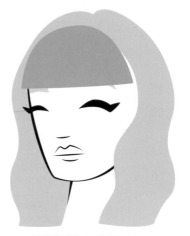

STRAIGHT BANGS

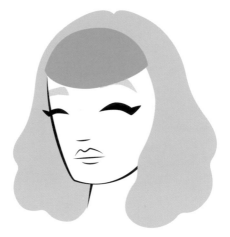

VINTAGE BANGS

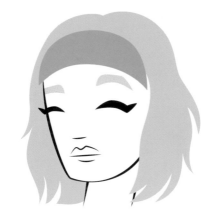

ARCHED BANGS

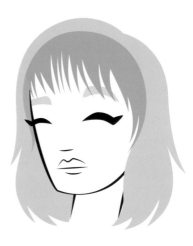

PIECEY BANGS

MORE BANG FOR YOUR BUCK

IT'S TRUE: KEEPING UP WITH BANGS REQUIRES PRETTY FREQUENT TRIMS. IF D.I.Y. IS TOO DAUNTING BUT THE PRICE OF CONSTANT HAIRCUTS IS EQUALLY SO, FEAR NOT! ASK YOUR STYLIST IF THEY OFFER SEPARATE PRICING FOR BANG TRIMS.

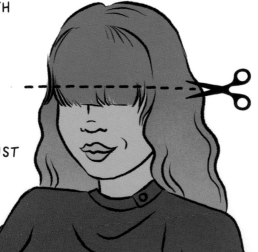

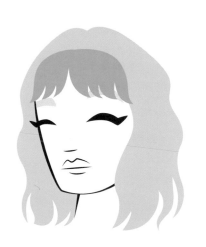

PARTED BANGS

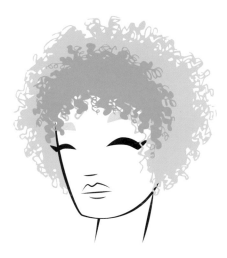

SHORT CURLY BANGS

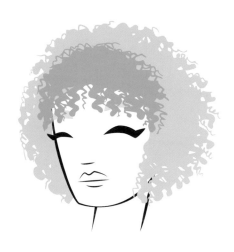

LONG CURLY BANGS

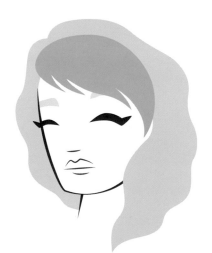

SIDESWEPT BANGS

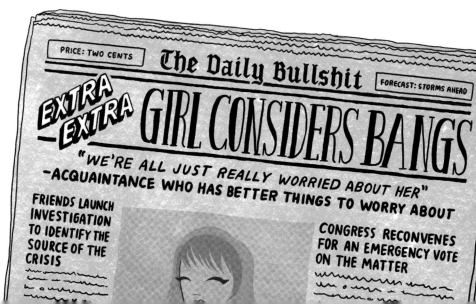

PRICE: TWO CENTS

The Daily Bullshit

FORECAST: STORMS AHEAD

EXTRA EXTRA GIRL CONSIDERS BANGS

"WE'RE ALL JUST REALLY WORRIED ABOUT HER"
–ACQUAINTANCE WHO HAS BETTER THINGS TO WORRY ABOUT

FRIENDS LAUNCH INVESTIGATION TO IDENTIFY THE SOURCE OF THE CRISIS

CONGRESS RECONVENES FOR AN EMERGENCY VOTE ON THE MATTER

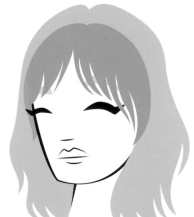

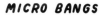
MICRO BANGS

ASYMMETRICAL BANGS

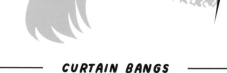
$\longleftarrow$ **CURTAIN BANGS** $\longrightarrow$

FEELIN' FRESH AS HELL

IF YOUR USUAL HAIR-WASHING ROUTINE IS NOT EVERY DAY, BUT YOUR NEW OILY BANGS HAVEN'T GOTTEN THE MEMO, DON'T SWEAT IT. LEAVE YOUR BANGS OUT OF YOUR SHOWER CAP TO SHAMPOO DURING YOUR DAILY SHOWER, OR EVEN WASH THEM OVER THE SINK WHEN YOU TAKE YOUR MAKEUP OFF AT NIGHT.

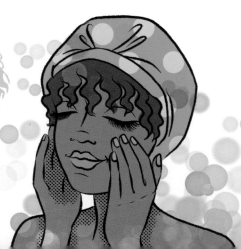

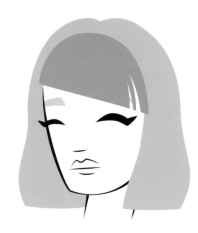

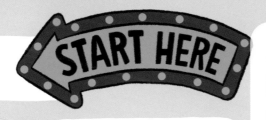
START HERE

SHOULD WE GET BACK TOGETHER?

IT'S NATURAL TO SECOND-GUESS YOUR DECISION A FEW (THOUSAND) TIMES AS YOU GRIEVE. AND SURE, MAYBE SOME TIME AND SPACE ARE ALL YOU NEEDED, BUT MORE OFTEN THAN NOT, THOSE IRRECONCILABLE DIFFERENCES WILL STILL BE WAITING FOR YOU IF YOU RETURN.

THINK ABOUT THE ISSUE THAT CAUSED THE BREAKUP. HAS THE STATUS OF THAT ISSUE CHANGED?

NO

NO, BUT I HAVE A NEW PERSPECTIVE ON IT

YES

ACTUALLY CHANGED OR ARE WE TALKING PROMISES?

PROMISES

ACTUALLY

HOW MANY TIMES HAVE YOU ALREADY BROKEN UP AND GOTTEN BACK TOGETHER?

2-200

NONE

HAVE YOU EVER HEARD AN ELDERLY COUPLE WHO IS RECOUNTING THEIR EPIC LOVE STORY SAY, "AND THEN WE BROKE UP, AND THEN GOT BACK TOGETHER (AND THEN BROKE UP AGAIN, AND THEN GOT BACK TOGETHER), AND THEN EVERYTHING WAS GREAT, AND WE'VE BEEN MARRIED 50 YEARS?"

YES

NO

YOU ARE LYING

OK NOW GO ASK YOUR BEST FRIEND.

SAID THEY WOULD KILL ME

SAID GO FOR IT!

GIRL NO

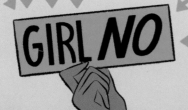

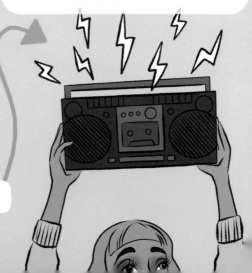

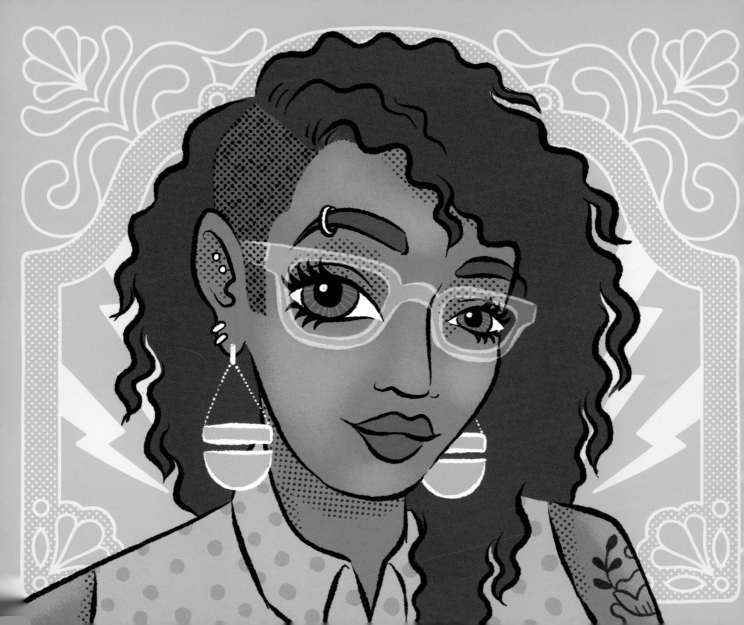

ON EDGE

UNDERCUTS AND SIDECUTS

BREAKUP HAIR IS ABOUT MAKING A CHANGE, BUT FOR YOU, MAYBE IT'S ALSO ABOUT MAKING A STATEMENT. IN THE PAST, PEOPLE MAY HAVE LABELED YOU AS THE AMIABLE, CAREFULLY COORDINATED, ALWAYS-PUNCTUAL TYPE. NOW THAT LIFE HAS HANDED YOU SOME HEARTBREAK, AND WITH IT A HEAPING DOSE OF CLARITY, YOU MAY FEEL LIKE MORE OF A "GET OUT OF MY WAY BECAUSE I'M A FORCE TO BE RECKONED WITH" TYPE. *AND YOU WANT THE WORLD TO KNOW IT.* GIRL, GET THE BUZZER OUT OF THAT BOX OF BULLSHIT YOUR EX LEFT BEHIND, BECAUSE UNDERCUTS AND SIDECUTS ARE THE PERFECT STYLE CHOICE FOR CONVEYING YOUR NEW TAKE-NO-SHIT TAKE ON LIFE.

UNDERCUTS

THE REAL BEAUTY OF UNDERCUTS IS THAT THEY ARE BASICALLY A BLANK CANVAS FOR WEARABLE ART. EVER WANTED A BADASS TATTOO, BUT LIKE, A MAGICAL ONE THAT FADES IN ABOUT TWO WEEKS? FRIEND, YOU HAVE FOUND IT. GET YOURSELF A STYLIST WHO KNOWS THEIR WAY AROUND WITH A BUZZER (TRY BARBERSHOPS), AND THE INTERNET WILL PROVIDE REFERENCE PHOTOS FOR EVERYTHING FROM DELICATE FLORAL MANDALAS TO A GODDAMN SLICE OF PIZZA. BE THE WEIRD ART THAT YOU (WE ALL) WISH TO SEE IN THE WORLD.

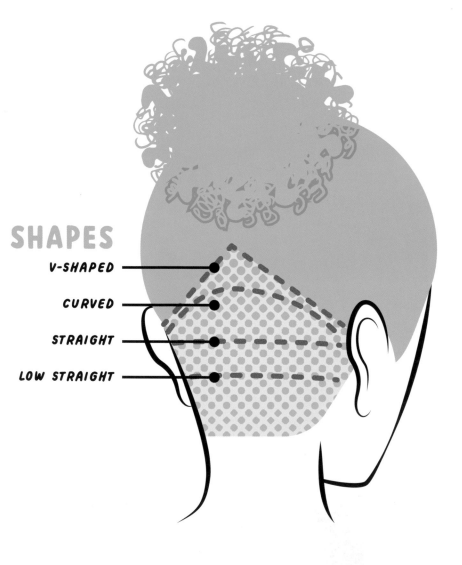

SHAPES

V-SHAPED

CURVED

STRAIGHT

LOW STRAIGHT

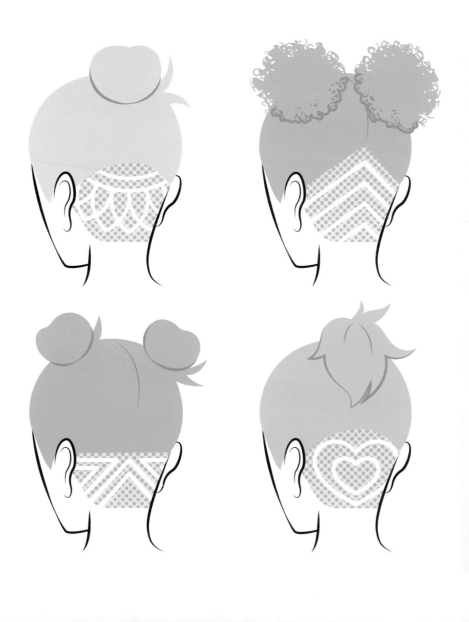

YOU'RE NEVER
TOO OLD TO
BREAK THE
RULES

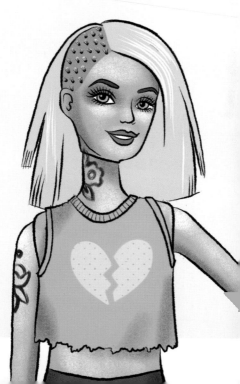

SIDECUTS

SOME MIGHT SAY THAT THIS TREND IS ALREADY OUT THE DOOR, BUT I'D LIKE TO THINK IT'S JUST GETTING STARTED. WHO DOESN'T LOVE AN ASYMMETRICAL LOOK? AND THIS IS ASYMMETRICAL VIBES *TO THE MAX*. ON THE SILVER SCREEN IT'S PRACTICALLY CODE FOR "HERE'S THE BADASS CHARACTER OF OUR STORY." AND IT HAS THAT SAME ENERGY IN REAL LIFE. WATCH OUT, WORLD: THIS CHICK WITH A SIDECUT IS HERE TO **GET SHIT DONE.**

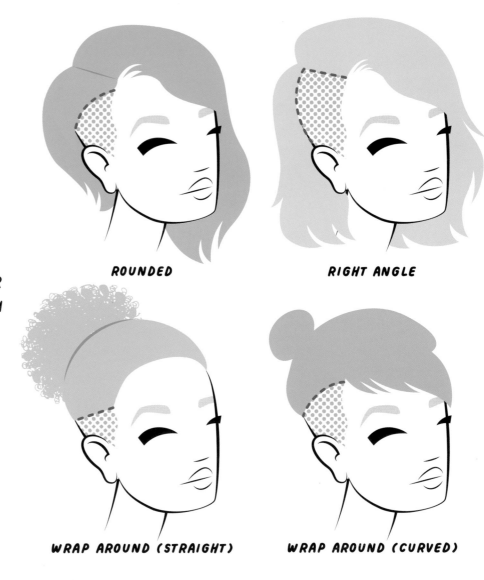

ROUNDED

RIGHT ANGLE

WRAP AROUND (STRAIGHT)

WRAP AROUND (CURVED)

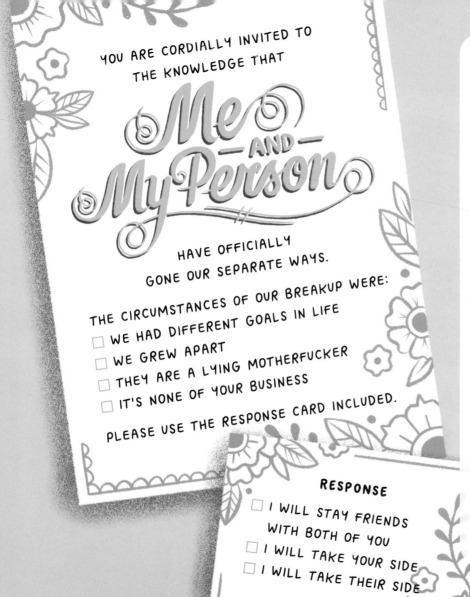

YOU ARE CORDIALLY INVITED TO THE KNOWLEDGE THAT

Me —AND— My Person

HAVE OFFICIALLY GONE OUR SEPARATE WAYS.

THE CIRCUMSTANCES OF OUR BREAKUP WERE:
- ☐ WE HAD DIFFERENT GOALS IN LIFE
- ☐ WE GREW APART
- ☐ THEY ARE A LYING MOTHERFUCKER
- ☐ IT'S NONE OF YOUR BUSINESS

PLEASE USE THE RESPONSE CARD INCLUDED.

RESPONSE
- ☐ I WILL STAY FRIENDS WITH BOTH OF YOU
- ☐ I WILL TAKE YOUR SIDE
- ☐ I WILL TAKE THEIR SIDE

THE ANNOUNCEMENT

ONE DREADED SIDE EFFECT OF BREAKING UP IS HAVING TO SPREAD THE NEWS. SURE, YOU'LL CALL YOUR MOM AND BEST FRIEND THE SAME DAY, IT WILL COME UP WITH COWORKERS THE SAME WEEK, BUT THEN THERE IS THE TRICKLE OF LESS FREQUENT INTERACTIONS WITH FRIENDS, ACQUAINTANCES, AND DISTANT RELATIVES WHO WILL ALL INEVITABLY ASK, "AND HOW IS 'SO-AND-SO' DOING?" *IF ONLY WE COULD JUST GET THIS ALL OVER WITH AT ONCE.*

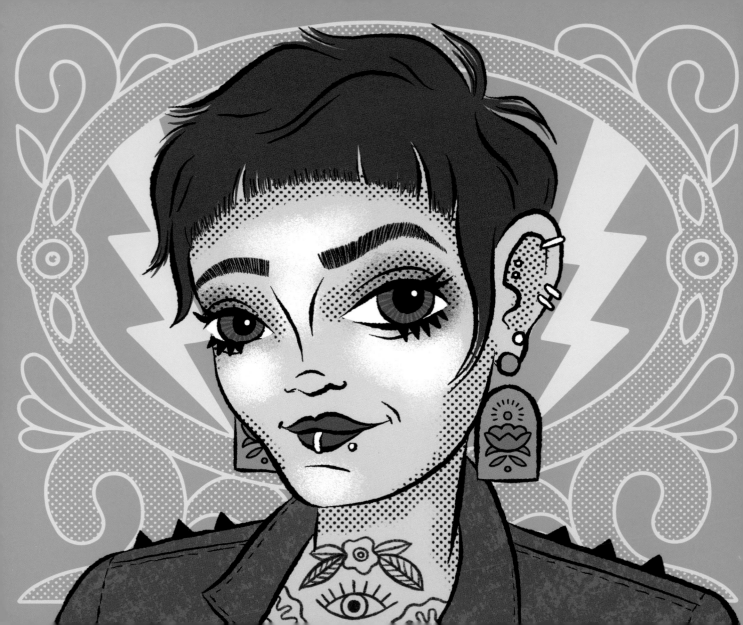

COMMITMENT ISSUES

PIXIES AND BUZZCUTS

LOOKING FOR A STYLE THAT WILL TURN HEADS AND, MORE IMPORTANTLY, MAKE JAWS DROP? GIRL, LET'S TALK ABOUT THE POWER OF PIXIES. CHOPPING OFF ALL OF YOUR HAIR IS AN ABSOLUTE POWER MOVE, A TOTAL MIDDLE FINGER TO SOCIETAL EXPECTATIONS. IT IS STRIKING, ON EVERY LEVEL. AND WHILE IT MIGHT SEEM SUDDEN TO OTHERS, IT'S PROBABLY NOT TO YOU. IF YOU'RE CONTEMPLATING A PIXIE NOW, YOU'VE PROBABLY WANTED ONE FOR A LONG TIME. THE ONLY DIFFERENCE IS THAT LATELY YOU'RE FUELED BY A BIT OF EXTRA POST-BREAKUP GUMPTION. ALREADY CALCULATING HOW LONG IT WILL TAKE TO GROW, IN THE EVENT YOU DON'T LIKE IT? IT'S TRUE: THERE'S NO GOING BACK (AT LEAST NOT IMMEDIATELY). YOU'RE IN IT FOR THE LONG HAUL. YOU MIGHT HAVE BEEN AFRAID OF COMMITMENT BEFORE, BUT NOW YOU'RE TAKING THE PLUNGE.

PIXIE 360

FOR PIXIE HAIRCUTS, YOU
DON'T JUST NEED REFERENCE
PHOTOS FOR WHAT THE
FRONT OF YOUR HAIR LOOKS
LIKE—YOU'LL NEED THE SIDES
AND BACK AS WELL. BROWSE
#PIXIE360 ON INSTAGRAM
TO GET ACQUAINTED WITH
A WORLD OF GLAMOROUS
OPTIONS.

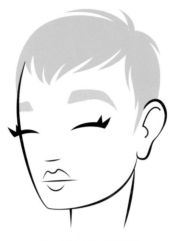

CLASSIC PIXIE

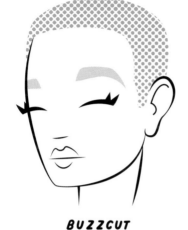

BUZZCUT

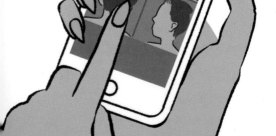

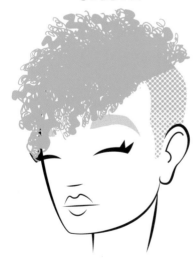

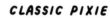

SIDESWEPT PIXIES

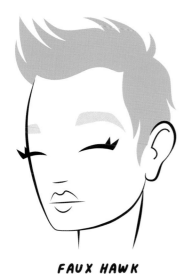

FAUX HAWK

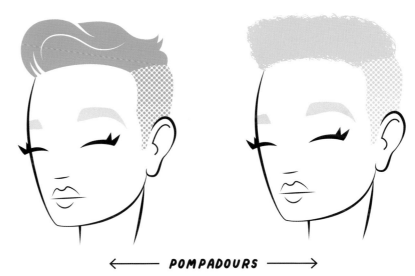

← **POMPADOURS** →

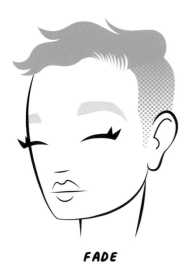

FADE

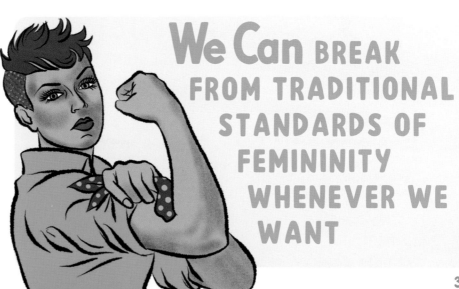

We Can BREAK FROM TRADITIONAL STANDARDS OF FEMININITY WHENEVER WE WANT

35

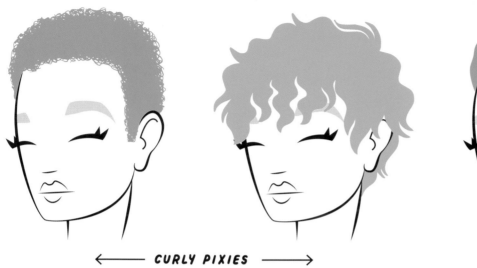

CURLY PIXIES

SLICKED BACK

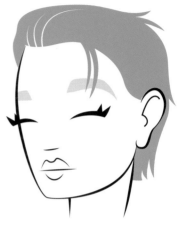

PRODUCT PSA

HAIR GEL KNOWS NO GENDER, AND "LADY" PRODUCTS ARE OFTEN PRICED HIGHER, SO FEEL FREE TO USE WHATEVER THE FUCK WORKS BEST FOR YOUR HAIR *AND YOUR BUDGET.*

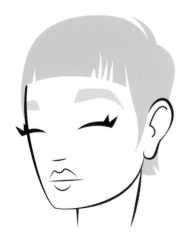

STRAIGHT BANG PIXIE

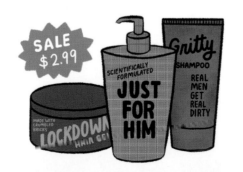

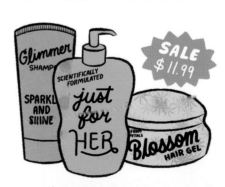

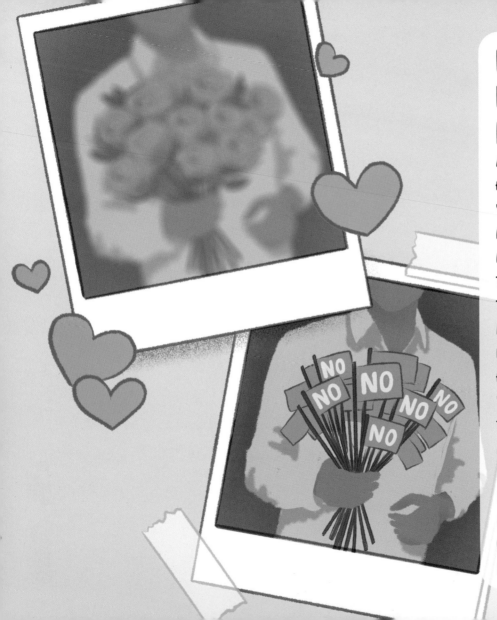

HINDSIGHT IS . . . A LITTLE FUZZY

AS YOUR RELATIONSHIP FADES INTO THE DISTANCE, YOUR RECOLLECTION OF IT MIGHT BECOME MORE AND MORE IDYLLIC, ADDING THE STING OF REGRET TO AN ALREADY PAINFUL PROCESS. BUT YOU ARE HERE FOR A REASON. FOCUS ON *THE FACTS* OF YOUR RELATIONSHIP, NOT THE FICTION THAT YOUR MEMORY IS CREATING. WHEN YOUR HEART DRIFTS INTO HAZY VISIONS OF HAPPIER TIMES, WAKE IT UP BY COUNTING ALL THOSE BRIGHT, CRISP RED FLAGS.

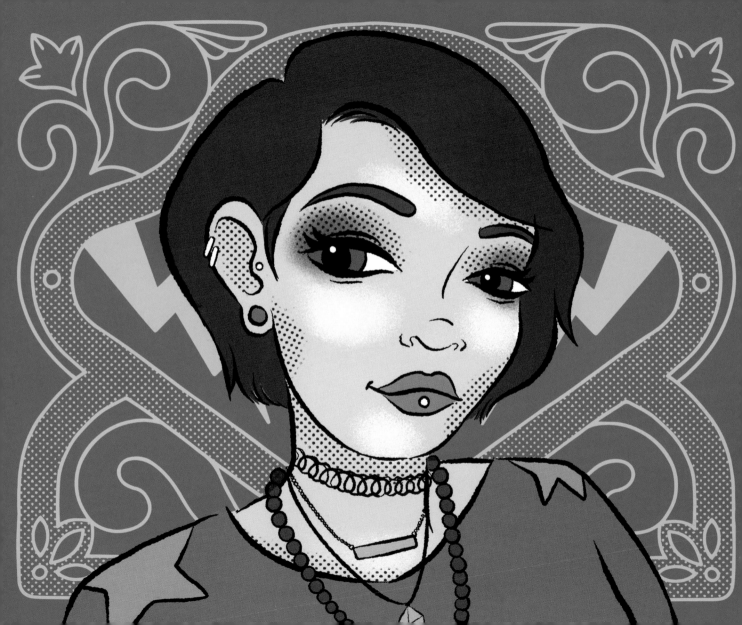

GROWING APART

GROWING OUT A PIXIE

IF YOU ALREADY HAVE A PIXIE HAIRCUT, IT MIGHT BE HARD TO ADMIT THAT YOU WANT TO GROW IT OUT. YOU'VE BEEN SUCH A CHAMPION FOR THE CAUSE OF SHORT HAIR! YOU PEP-TALKED EVERY WOMAN WHO SAID, "I JUST WISH I COULD PULL THAT OFF," YOU SASSED ANYONE WHO DARED IMPLY THAT IT COULD AFFECT ONE'S DATING PROSPECTS, AND YOUR STYLING TUTORIAL VIDEOS HAVE, WELL, QUITE A FEW FOLLOWERS. AFTER ALL THAT, LEAVING THE PIXIE CLUB NOW FEELS LIKE YOU'RE BETRAYING SOMETHING. BUT REMEMBER THAT BREAKUP HAIR IS ABOUT WHAT *YOU* WANT. AND RIGHT NOW, YOU WANT SOME SPACE TO GROW, TO CHANGE, AND MAYBE SOME LENGTH TO TRY OUT OMBRÉ. YOU HAVE AS MUCH OF A RIGHT TO GET A RETRO BOB AS THE NEXT GAL, AND YOU'RE GOING TO ROCK IT.

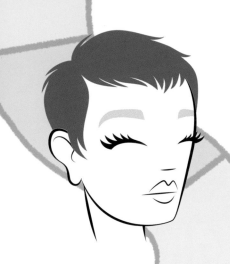

THIS JOURNEY IS NOT FOR THE FAINT OF HEART

GROWING OUT YOUR HAIR CAN FEEL A BIT LIKE TORTURE IF YOU'RE USED TO FRESH CUTS AND FRESH COMPLIMENTS ON A REGULAR BASIS. BUT YOU CAN DO THIS! REWARD YOURSELF ALONG THE WAY, STAY STRONG, AND MAYBE HIDE ANY SCISSORS THAT COULD BE USED FOR A LATE-NIGHT PIXIE RESTORATION.

THE DECISION
FIRST MONTH

YOU HAVE RESOLVED TO START THIS MARATHON, TO FINALLY GROW OUT YOUR HAIR. YOU HELD A PRESS CONFERENCE AND RALLIED SUPPORTERS. YOU FEEL GREAT ABOUT IT, BUT SO FAR IT'S ALL TALK, NO ACTION.

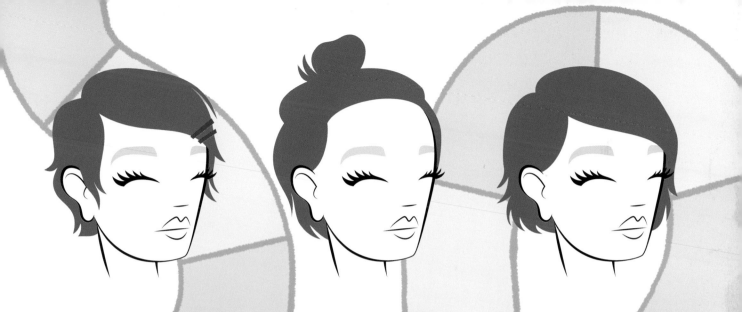

THE INDECISION
2 MONTHS

YOU DO NOT FEEL GREAT ABOUT IT. YOU LOOK SORELY OVERDUE FOR A HAIRCUT, AND IT WILL REQUIRE EVERY BIT OF RESTRAINT YOU POSSESS TO NOT RUN TO THE NEAREST SALON FOR A TRIM.

THE TORMENT
4 MONTHS

DESPITE YOUR DILIGENT EFFORTS TO RESHAPE THE LAYERS AS THEY GROW AND A WHOLE NEW PLETHORA OF HAIR ACCESSORIES, YOU'RE FAR FROM LOOKING LIKE YOU GOT THIS HAIRSTYLE ON PURPOSE.

THE "MEH" TIMES
6 MONTHS

YOU NO LONGER LOOK LIKE YOU'VE BEEN STRANDED ON AN ISLAND, WITHOUT ACCESS TO FOOD OR WATER OR PROPER HAIRCUTS. YOU'RE AT A LENGTH THAT'S NOT IDEAL, BUT NOT INSUFFERABLE.

41

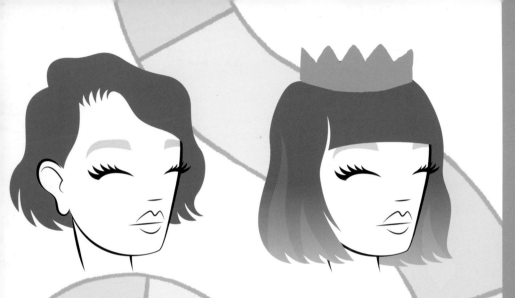

END IN SIGHT

7-10 MONTHS

YOU ARE SOOOOO CLOSE TO YOUR DREAM HAIRCUT. JUST KEEP YOUR EYE ON THE PRIZE, AND KEEP BUILDING THAT HAIR INSPO BOARD UNTIL YOU CAN AUTHOR AN ENCYCLOPEDIC GUIDE TO BLUNT BANGS.

FINISH LINE

YOU MADE IT! CELEBRATE WITH CHAMPAGNE AND AN HBO SUBSCRIPTION. THIS IS A TRIUMPH THAT FEW WILL UNDERSTAND THE GRAVITY OF, BUT *YOU* KNOW THAT YOU HAVE JUST DISPLAYED PATIENCE OF OLYMPIC PROPORTIONS.

THE SECRET TO GROWING YOUR HAIR OUT IS: HAIRCUTS

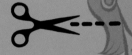

AS YOUR HAIR GROWS, IT ALSO NEEDS RESHAPING. TRIMMING BACK THAT BOTTOM LAYER, UNTIL THE TOP LAYER CATCHES UP WITH IT, IS CRUCIAL. IT'S TEMPTING TO KEEP IT BECAUSE YOU CAN CLEARLY SEE THE PROGRESS, BUT UNLESS YOU'RE READY TO ROCK A MULLET, GIRL, THAT LAYER NEEDS TO GO.

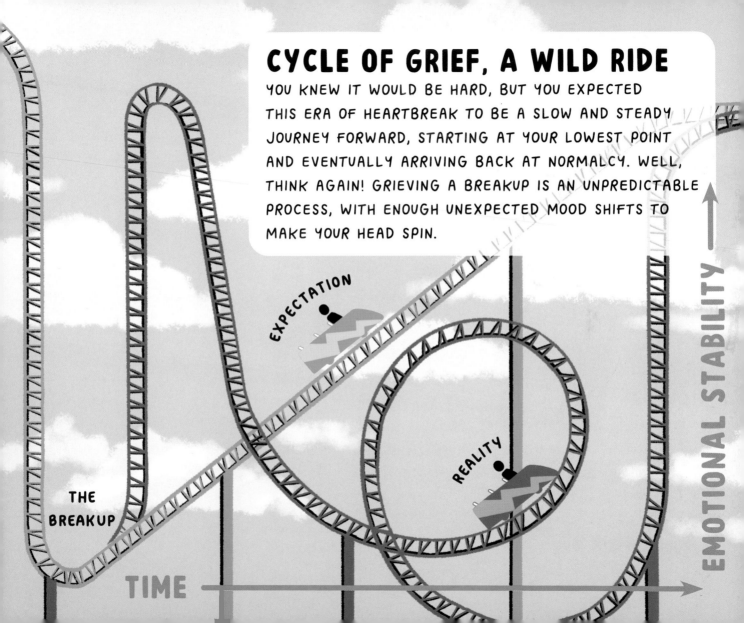

CYCLE OF GRIEF, A WILD RIDE

YOU KNEW IT WOULD BE HARD, BUT YOU EXPECTED THIS ERA OF HEARTBREAK TO BE A SLOW AND STEADY JOURNEY FORWARD, STARTING AT YOUR LOWEST POINT AND EVENTUALLY ARRIVING BACK AT NORMALCY. WELL, THINK AGAIN! GRIEVING A BREAKUP IS AN UNPREDICTABLE PROCESS, WITH ENOUGH UNEXPECTED MOOD SHIFTS TO MAKE YOUR HEAD SPIN.

EXPECTATION

REALITY

THE BREAKUP

TIME

EMOTIONAL STABILITY

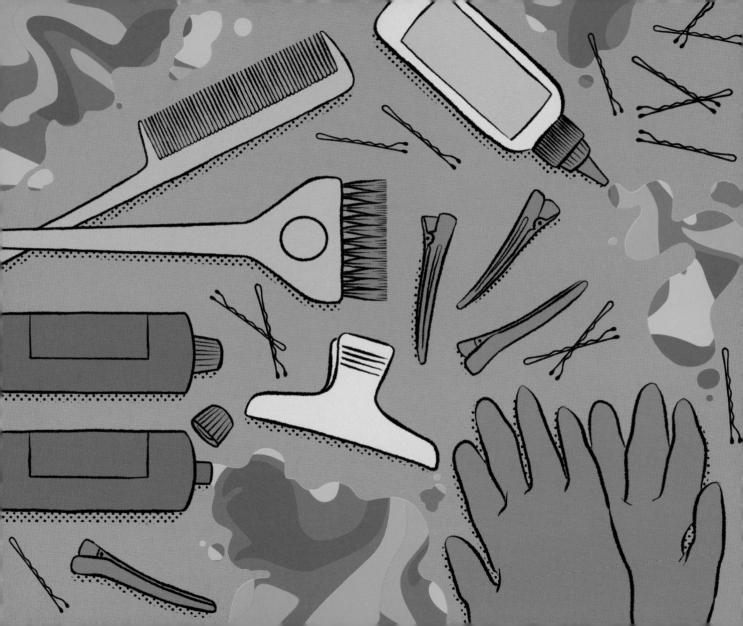

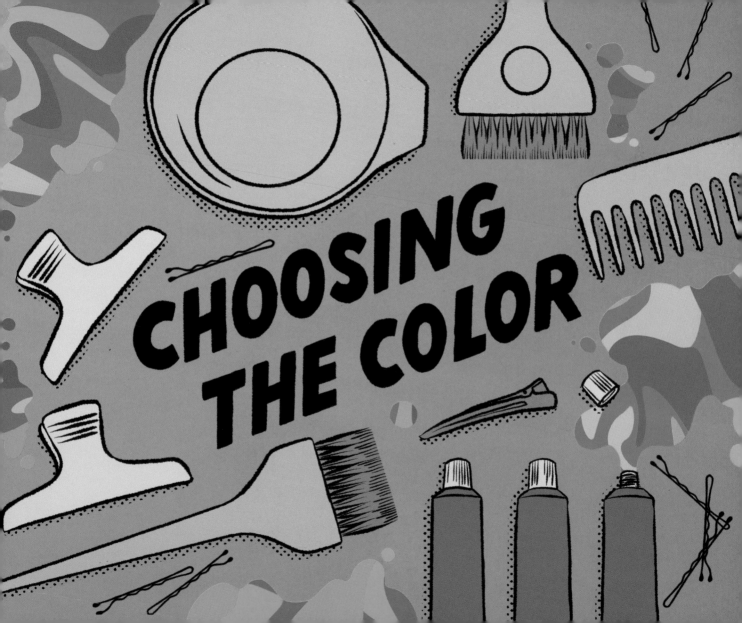

CHOOSING THE COLOR

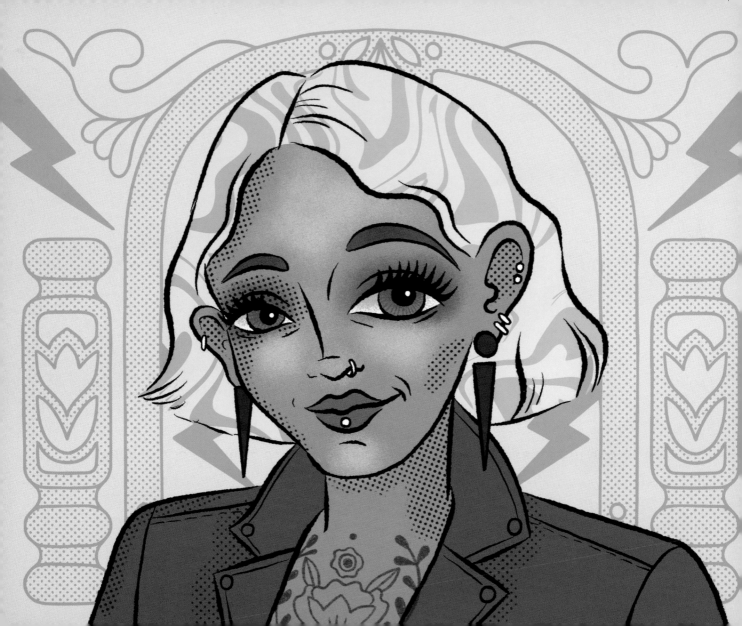

FRESH START

GOING LIGHTER

LIGHTENING YOUR HAIR IS A RISKY MOVE, BUT YOU MIGHT BE DOWN FOR RISKS THESE DAYS. SOMEONE IS BOUND TO GIVE YOU AN EARFUL ABOUT HOW IT'S GOING TO BE SO MUCH UPKEEP, YOUR HAIR IS GOING TO FEEL MORE DAMAGED, AND, SURE, THERE ARE A MILLION GOOD REASONS FOR WHY YOU SHOULD PLAY IT SAFE. YOU COULD ALSO WEAR SENSIBLE SHOES, CUT COUPONS, AND AVOID DRIVING AFTER DARK. BUT YOU'VE JUST HAD YOUR HEART BROKEN—NOW IS NOT THE TIME TO THINK ABOUT FUTURE PLANS (OR FUTURE ROOT TOUCH-UPS). RIGHT NOW, YOU NEED TO BUY THAT OVERPRICED LEATHER JACKET, GO OUT DANCING UNTIL THE BARS CLOSE, AND DYE YOUR HAIR FUCKING PLATINUM.

LIGHTER

DARKER

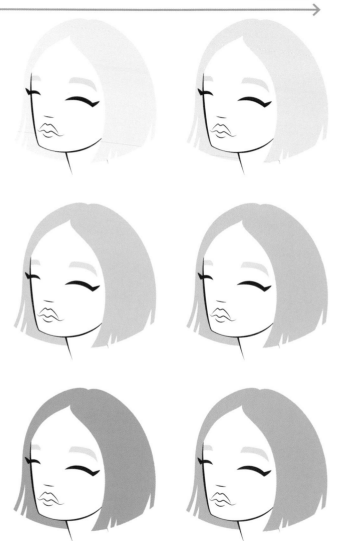

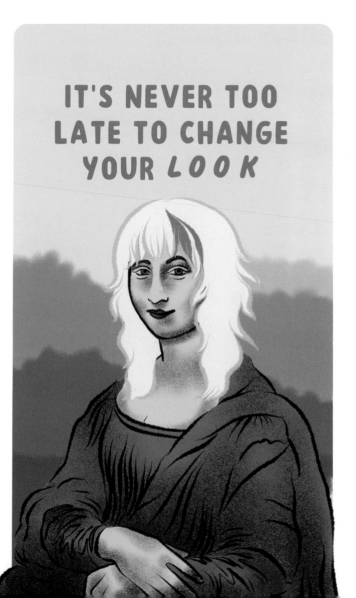

IT'S NEVER TOO LATE TO CHANGE YOUR *LOOK*

DRINK UP!

WHATEVER THE CIRCUMSTANCES OF YOUR BREAKUP WERE, GIRL, I'M GOING TO GUESS YOU NEED A STRONG DRINK. FOLLOW THESE FUN COCKTAIL RECIPES AS YOU CONTINUE ON YOUR PATH TOWARD HEALTH AND HEALING.

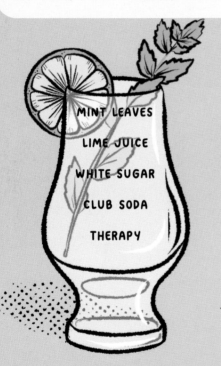

MINT LEAVES

LIME JUICE

WHITE SUGAR

CLUB SODA

THERAPY

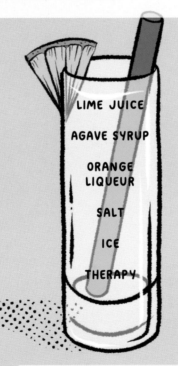

LIME JUICE

AGAVE SYRUP

ORANGE LIQUEUR

SALT

ICE

THERAPY

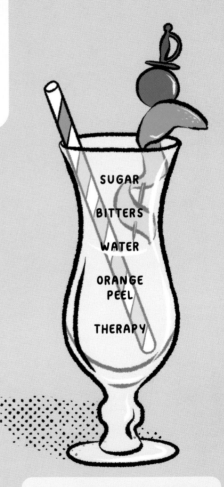

SUGAR

BITTERS

WATER

ORANGE PEEL

THERAPY

THEY BROKE UP WITH YOU VIA TEXT

YOU BROKE UP WITH *THEM* VIA A MYSTERIOUS NOTE AND SKIPPING TOWN

YOU FINALLY ACKNOWLEDGED THE ISSUES YOUR SISTER POINTED OUT ON DAY ONE

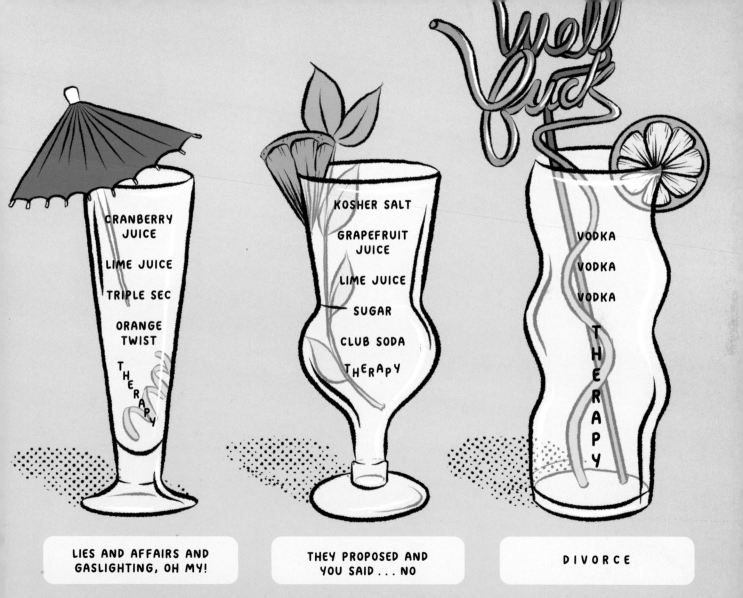

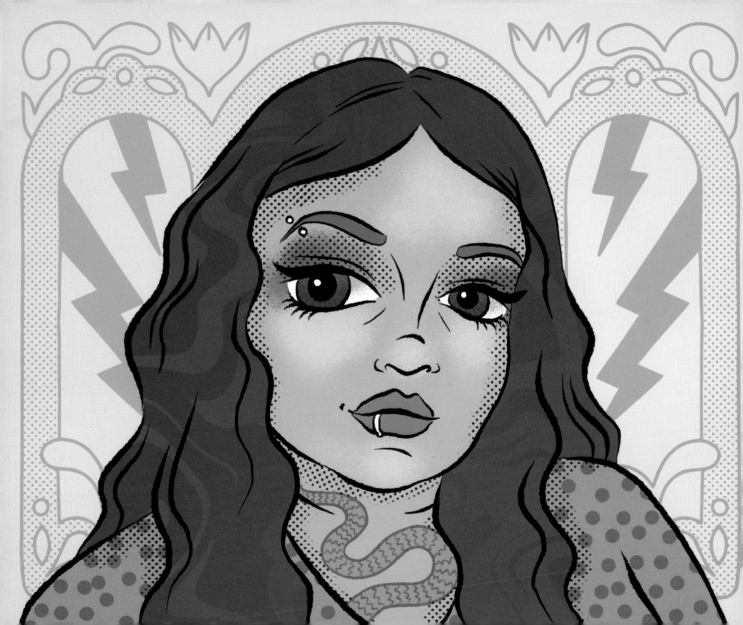

NEXT LEVEL
GOING DARKER

YOU'VE SUCCESSFULLY EMERGED FROM THE "DRINKING WINE IN BED" PHASE OF HEARTBREAK AND ARE WELL INTO THE SELF-IMPROVEMENT KICK. YOU'RE JOGGING, MEDITATING, WAKING UP EARLIER, DOING A SOCIAL MEDIA CLEANSE, READING MEMOIRS, LEARNING WATERCOLOR. AND YOU'RE LOOKING FOR THE PERFECT HAIR CHANGE THAT CAPTURES THE "NEW AND IMPROVED" YOU. GOING A FEW SHADES DARKER THAN YOUR NATURAL HAIR CAN FEEL LIKE YOU'RE STEPPING INTO AN OLDER, WISER VERSION OF YOURSELF. WITH A LOOK THAT SPEAKS TO THIS NEWLY BALANCED, CULTURED, VEGETABLE-EATING SELF, YOU MIGHT START REGAINING THE CONFIDENCE YOU NEED TO GO OUT INTO THE WORLD, JOIN A BOOK CLUB, TAKE YOUR DOG TO THE PARK, AND DELETE YOUR EX'S NUMBER.

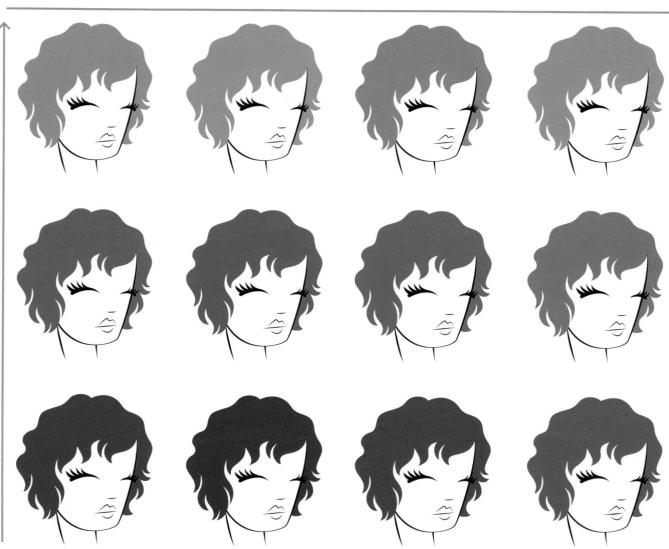

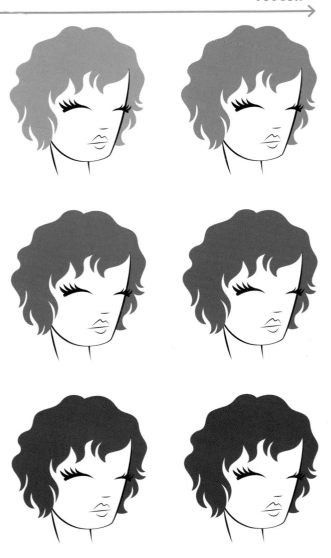

HAIRSTYLISTS ARE THE HEROES WE DON'T DESERVE

IN THIS TIME OF TRANSFORMATION, YOUR STYLIST IS YOUR SPIRIT GUIDE, YOUR ACCESS TO THE WORLD BEYOND. SO TREAT THEM WELL. STYLISTS SPEND YEARS LEARNING THEIR CRAFT, THEY ARE PASSIONATE CREATIVES, THEY KINDLY LISTEN TO OUR BULLSHIT (I MEAN LOVE LIVES) FOR HOURS. AND YET THEY RARELY GET THE STABILITY OF A SALARY, P.T.O., OR SICK TIME AND ARE ON THEIR FEET ALL DAY. THEY DESERVE THE WORLD AND THEN SOME— THE LEAST WE CAN DO IS GIVE A GOOD TIP.

THE UNIVERSE KNOWS BEST

LETTING GO OF YOUR PAST RELATIONSHIP WILL INEVITABLY LEAD YOU TO WONDER ABOUT THE FUTURE. AND WHEN IT COMES TO FINDING (AND KEEPING) LOVE, WE ALL KNOW WHERE TO LOOK FOR ANSWERS. OBVIOUSLY, IT'S FATE. COINCIDENCE. LUCK. STARS ALIGNING. SO, TO DETERMINE NEXT STEPS, AWAY FROM HEARTBREAK AND TOWARD SOULMATED BLISS, LET'S CONSULT THE DIVINE TO REVEAL YOUR ROMANTIC DESTINY.

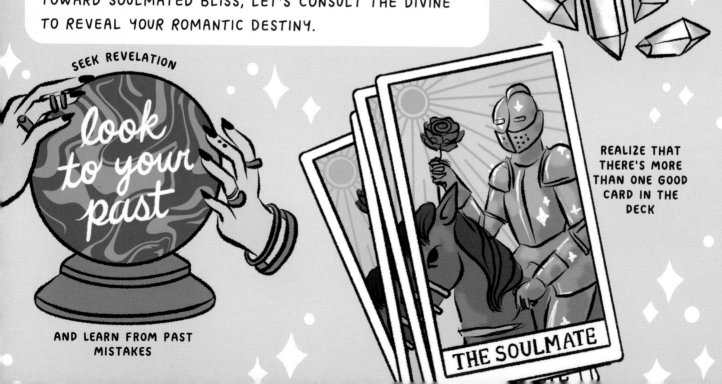

HEAL YOURSELF FIRST

SEEK REVELATION

look to your past

AND LEARN FROM PAST MISTAKES

REALIZE THAT THERE'S MORE THAN ONE GOOD CARD IN THE DECK

THE SOULMATE

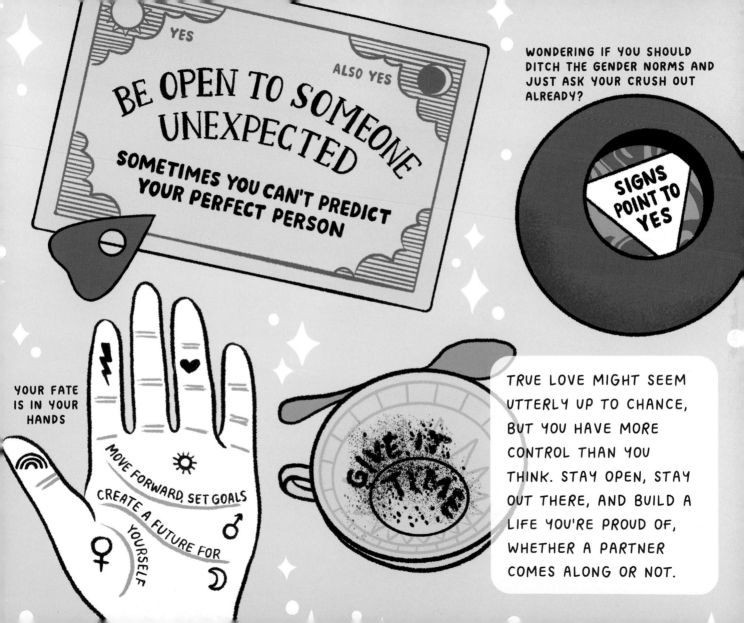

YES

ALSO YES

BE OPEN TO SOMEONE UNEXPECTED

SOMETIMES YOU CAN'T PREDICT YOUR PERFECT PERSON

WONDERING IF YOU SHOULD DITCH THE GENDER NORMS AND JUST ASK YOUR CRUSH OUT ALREADY?

SIGNS POINT TO YES

YOUR FATE IS IN YOUR HANDS

MOVE FORWARD, SET GOALS

CREATE A FUTURE FOR YOURSELF

GIVE IT TIME

TRUE LOVE MIGHT SEEM UTTERLY UP TO CHANCE, BUT YOU HAVE MORE CONTROL THAN YOU THINK. STAY OPEN, STAY OUT THERE, AND BUILD A LIFE YOU'RE PROUD OF, WHETHER A PARTNER COMES ALONG OR NOT.

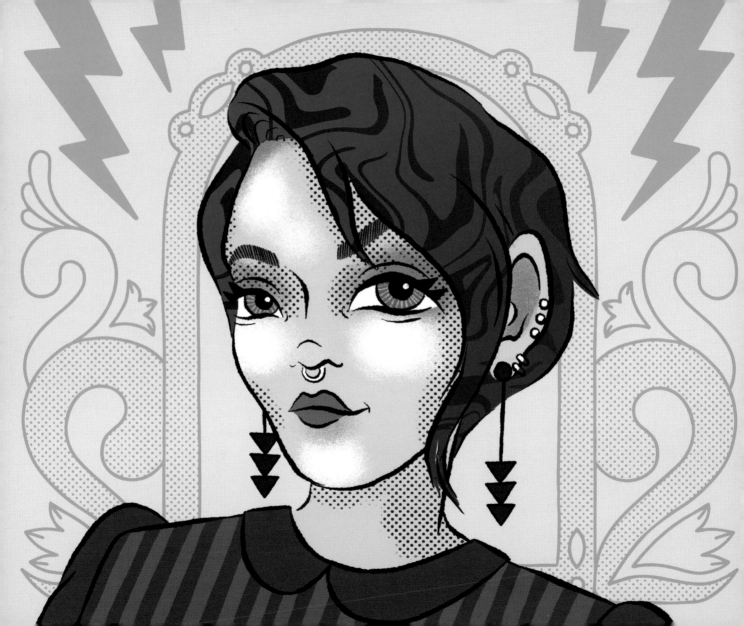

NEW FLAME

REDS

FEW WOMEN CHOOSE RED AS THEIR LONG-TERM HAIR COLOR, BUT WE ALL HAVE TO TRY IT ONCE. JUST LIKE THAT NEW HOTTIE YOU'RE SEEING, IT PROBABLY WON'T LAST LONG, BUT THAT DOESN'T MEAN IT'S NOT A PERFECT FIT FOR YOU RIGHT NOW. YOU'RE LIVING IN THE MOMENT, EXPERIMENTING WITH A NEW SENSE OF SELF. YOU'RE TAKING SWING-DANCING LESSONS, TRYING YOUR HAND AT PHOTOGRAPHY, COOKING WITH SPICES YOU'VE NEVER HEARD OF. YOU MIGHT EVEN BE *GASP* ONLINE DATING. NOT EVERYTHING FROM THIS PHASE OF LIFE IS GOING TO STICK, BUT YOU'RE ALONG FOR THE RIDE. YOU DESERVE A LITTLE FLING, HAIR-WISE AND OTHERWISE.

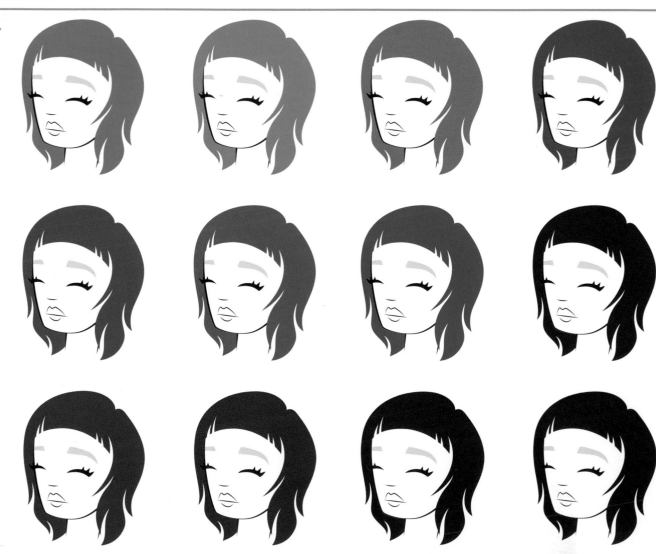

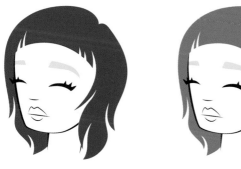

COOLER →

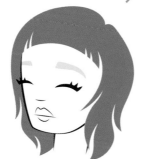
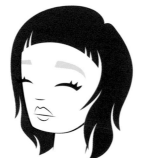
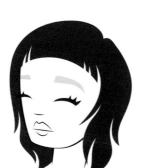
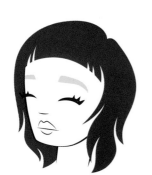

LOVE YOUR HAIR HISTORY

FOR ALL THE PROGRESS WE'VE MADE TOWARD SELF-LOVE IN THE HERE AND NOW, WE HAVE A WAYS TO GO WHEN IT COMES TO NOT HATING ON OUR PAST SELVES, ESPECIALLY OUR HAIR. WE RECOIL AT PICTURES OF HIGH SCHOOL AND TRY TO ERASE ANY RECORD OF OUR FASHION SENSE A DECADE AGO. INSTEAD OF CRINGING, LET'S CELEBRATE OUR JOURNEYS OF SELF-EXPRESSION. I BET YOU (AND YOUR SCENE-STER KID MULLET) WERE ACTUALLY PRETTY AWESOME BACK IN THE DAY.

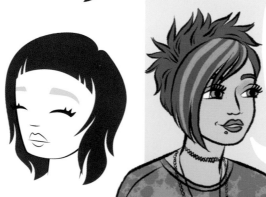
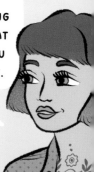

I KNOW IT WAS THE EARLY 2000S, AND YOU WERE BEING PRETTY FASHION-FORWARD AT THE TIME, AND I ACCEPT YOU *AND ADMIRE YOU* FOR THAT.

I MEAN, DUDE, YOUR HAIR IS PRETTY WEIRD TOO.

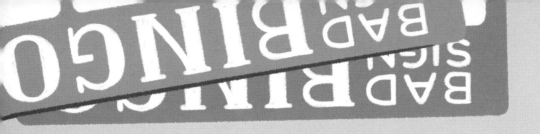

TO THE LEFT, TO THE LEFT (SWIPE)

LIST THE REASONS YOU'RE ABOVE IT ALL DAMN DAY—SOONER OR LATER YOU *WILL* DOWNLOAD DATING APPS. A GOOD CATCH IS RARE, AND SWIPING THROUGH THE NO'S CAN BE EXHAUSTING, SO YOU MIGHT AS WELL MAKE A GAME OF IT! GATHER YOUR FELLOW SINGLE FRIENDS AND GET READY FOR SOME NOT-SO-OLD-FASHIONED BINGO.

BAD SIGN BINGO

MATCHING OUTFITS WITH SIBLINGS	USING THE PROFILE TO ADVERTISE THEIR BUSINESS	OBVIOUS PIC WITH AN EX-GIRLFRIEND	THE "NOT MY KID" BIO	ALREADY SEEMS MAD AT YOU
"JUST LOVES ADVENTURES!"	PROUDLY POSING WITH A DEAD ANIMAL	CASUALLY HANGING OUT ON A YACHT	NOTHING BUT SELFIES	LISTS BAD SONG LYRICS AS MOTTO FOR LIFE
NOTHING BUT GROUP PICTURES	WEARING SUNGLASSES IN EVERY PIC	FREE	ALL THE PICS ARE TRAVEL BRAGS	IS THIS A DATING BIO OR A RÉSUMÉ?
COUPLE SEEKING A THREESOME	USES BIO TO DESCRIBE THEIR "TYPE"	LISTS THEIR HEIGHT AND/OR WEIGHT	"I DON'T CHECK THIS APP MUCH, JUST DM ME"	HAS THE SAME NAME AS YOUR PARENT
CROSSES OTHER FACES OUT OF PICS LIKE A PSYCHO	CAN I JUST DATE THIS DOG?	JUST THE CREEPIEST CREEPER WHO EVER CREEPED	TOTALLY LYING ABOUT THEIR AGE	PROUDLY POSING WITH A WEAPON

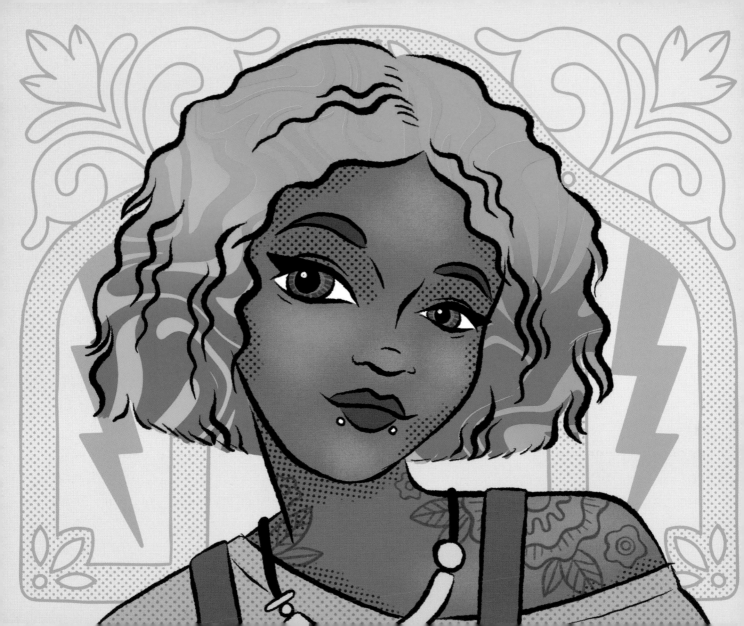

BRIGHT SIDE

BRIGHTS

IT HAS BEEN A ROUGH BOUT OF HEARTACHE, BUT THE CLOUDS ARE FINALLY PARTING AND YOU CAN SEE THE SUN AGAIN. NOW THAT THE WORST OF IT IS OVER, THINGS ARE FINALLY LOOKING UP. THE GRASS SEEMS GREENER, ROSES REDDER, AND PUPPIES ARE EVEN CUTER. YOU'RE SINGING LOUDLY WITH THE RADIO, SPENDING TIME OUTDOORS, AND MAKING NEW FRIENDS. YOU WANT A NEW LOOK, NOT BECAUSE YOU'RE STILL SAD, BUT BECAUSE YOU'RE FINALLY HEALING. YOU'VE ALWAYS MARVELED AT THOSE NEON HAIR COLORS BUT DIDN'T THINK YOU COULD EMBODY THAT KIND OF ENERGY. BUT NOW THAT THE DARK DAYS ARE BEHIND YOU, THIS NEW LIFE IS ELECTRIC, AND YOU WANT TO LOOK AS VIBRANT AS YOU FEEL.

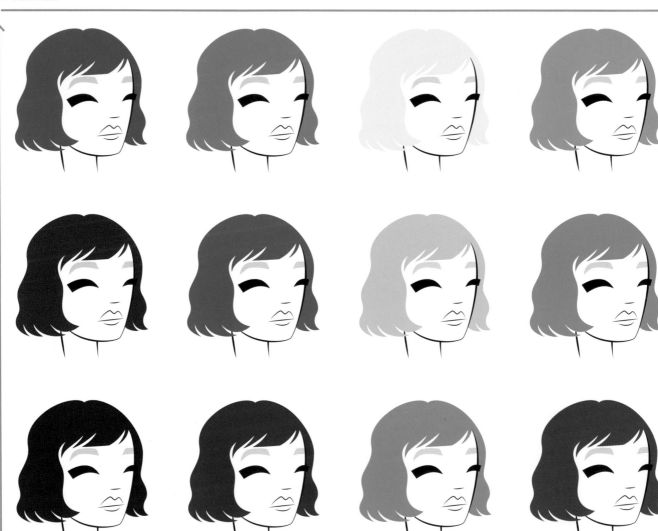

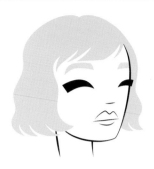

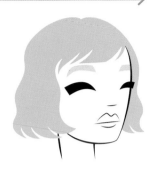

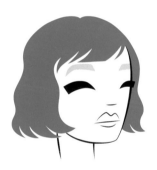

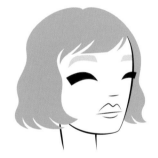

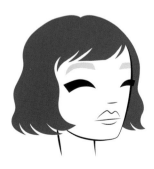

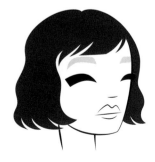

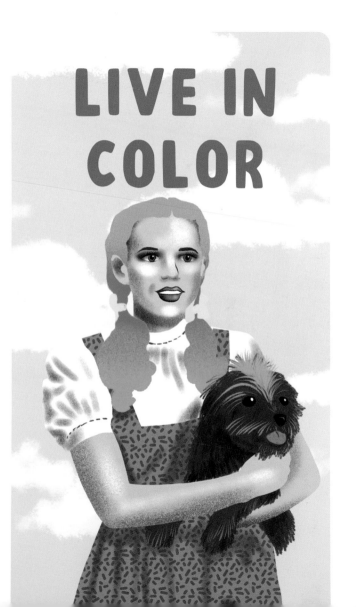

LIVE IN COLOR

AFTER A BREAKUP, IT'S EASY TO FEEL LIKE A FAILURE. BUT IN REALITY, EXITING A RELATIONSHIP THAT JUST WASN'T RIGHT, THAT TOOK HARD FUCKING WORK. MAYBE THE SPLIT WAS AS CLEAR-CUT AS KICKING THEIR CHEATING ASS OUT THE DOOR. MAYBE IT WAS A MUTUAL SOB-FEST AND TOOK HOURS OF TALKING. WHATEVER YOUR BREAKUP LOOKED LIKE, WHAT CAME BEFORE IT WAS A MARATHON OF DIFFICULT COMMUNICATION, SELF-REFLECTION, AND SHEER WILLPOWER TO GET YOU TO THAT DECISION. YOU DESERVE TO SEE YOURSELF NOT AS A QUITTER BUT AS A CHAMP WHO FINISHED ONE HELL OF A RACE.

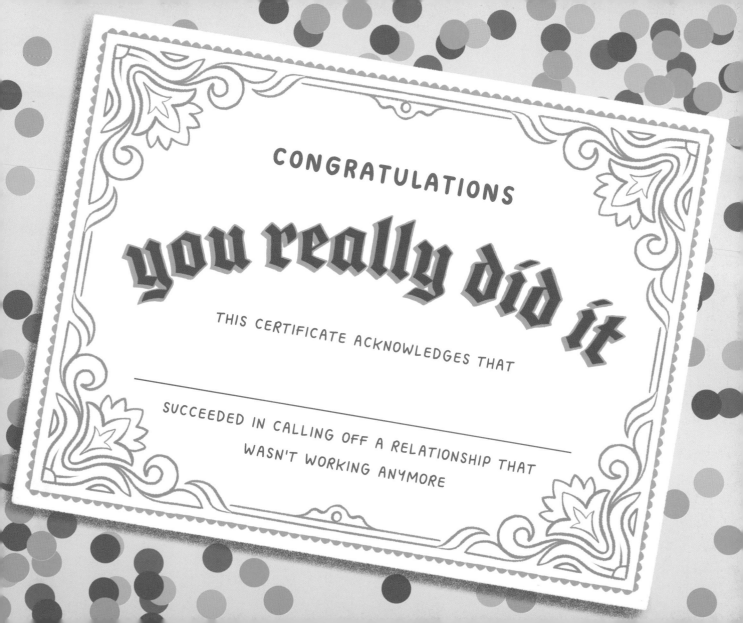

CONGRATULATIONS

you really did it

THIS CERTIFICATE ACKNOWLEDGES THAT

_____

SUCCEEDED IN CALLING OFF A RELATIONSHIP THAT
WASN'T WORKING ANYMORE

AT THE HEART OF IT

EXPLORING AND DEFINING YOUR STYLE ISN'T SILLY OR VAIN. IT'S ABOUT GETTING TO KNOW YOURSELF. AND AFTER A BREAKUP, YOU'RE HAVING TO DO THAT ALL OVER AGAIN. OF COURSE, A NEW HAIRSTYLE WON'T HEAL YOU. NEITHER WILL A NEW WARDROBE, A NEW TATTOO, OR A NEW PUPPY (ACTUALLY, A PUPPY MIGHT). HEARTBREAK IS SOME REAL SHIT, AND NO MATTER HOW MANY HAIRSTYLES YOU TRY, SELF-HELP BOOKS YOU READ, OR TAROT CARD READINGS YOU GET, YOU CANNOT RUSH THE ONE THING THAT DOES HEAL: TIME.

(BUT, LIKE, TOTALLY STILL GET THAT PIXIE CUT.)

ACKNOWLEDGMENTS

THE FIRST PERSON I ABSOLUTELY MUST THANK IS MY
FRIEND AND FELLOW ASPIRING WRITER LAUREN DODGE.
SHE HAS BEEN MY UNOFFICIAL EDITOR FOR THIS PROJECT
LONG BEFORE I HAD AN AGENT OR A BOOK DEAL—SHE HAS
READ ALMOST EVERY DRAFT AND TALKED ME THROUGH
EVERY MAJOR CONTENT CHANGE. LAUREN, YOU ARE AN
ALL-STAR! ANOTHER MAJOR THANKS IS DUE TO MY AGENT,
DANIELLE CHIOTTI—I'M NOT SURE I BELIEVED THIS BOOK
WAS ACTUALLY GOING TO HAPPEN UNTIL YOU CAME ON
BOARD—A REAL-LIFE PROFESSIONAL PUBLISHING-WORLD
PERSON, AND YOU SOLD THE HELL OUT OF IT. AND A HUGE
AND ETERNAL THANK-YOU TO MY LOVE, COLIN AVERILL,
WHO SUPPORTED US WHILE I FINISHED THIS BOOK.

THANK YOU, MATTHEW HAGERMAN, FOR ALWAYS BEING
MY CREATIVE BRAINSTORMING BUDDY AND VICTORIO
MARASIGAN FOR BEING THE MOST WONDERFULLY DETAIL-
ORIENTED REVIEWER—YOUR NOTES WERE MY BIBLE.
THANK YOU TO ALL MY FRIENDS WHO READ A DRAFT

SOMEWHERE ALONG THE WAY AND HELPED ME MAKE IT BETTER. KRISTEN MAZZAFERRO, TAYLOR BRADBURY, AMANDA HERRERA, MICHELLE AYOUBI, HANNAH AYOUBI, JOSH HEINLEIN, SARAH WARREN, AND WHOMEVER ELSE I DRAGGED INTO THIS, THANK YOU ALL. THANK YOU TO MY DESIGN MENTOR, DAVID STEADMAN—I AM ASHAMED TO SAY I DIDN'T EVEN KNOW HOW TO PROPERLY SET UP A GODDAMN PAGE GRID BEFORE YOU HIRED ME, AND THIS BOOK WOULDN'T BE HALF AS GOOD WITHOUT THE DESIGN EXPERTISE I'VE GLEANED FROM YOU OVER THE YEARS.

THANK YOU TO BRITT WARREN, MY BEST FRIEND, WHO HAS TALKED ME THROUGH ALL MY BIG HAIR DECISIONS (AND RELATIONSHIP DECISIONS) OF THE PAST DECADE. I WOULD NOT BE THIS INTO HAIR IF I DIDN'T HAVE SOMEONE TO SHARE MY OBSESSION WITH.

THANK YOU TO MY MOTHER, WHO DOES NOT LIKE THE WORD "FEMINISM," BUT NEVERTHELESS RAISED ME TO BELIEVE THAT I CAN DO ANYTHING, THAT I AM WORTHY OF EVERYTHING, AND THAT NO MATTER WHAT I LOOK LIKE, I AM **HOT SHIT**.

ABOUT THE AUTHOR

JENNA LUECKE TAKES HER COFFEE BLACK, LIVES FOR TRUE CRIME PODCASTS, DYES HER HAIR WITH ARCTIC FOX'S *SUNSET ORANGE*, ONLY HAS TWO EXES (BUT WENT THROUGH SIX BREAKUPS BETWEEN THEM), HAS ALWAYS, *ALWAYS* WANTED TO BE AN ARTIST, AND NEVER PLANNED ON BEING AN AUTHOR. BUT AFTER A DEGREE IN DESIGN, A LIFETIME OF SKETCHBOOKS, AND ONE BIG OL' HEARTBREAK, THIS BOOK JUST KIND OF APPEARED.

WHILE NOT AN EXPERT ON HAIR IN THE TRADITIONAL SENSE, JENNA HAS TRIED THE MAJORITY OF HAIRCUTS DISCUSSED IN THIS BOOK, GONE THROUGH A RAINBOW OF HAIR DYES, AND KNOWS FROM EXPERIENCE TO JUST *GET THE DAMN BANGS*.

JENNA LUECKE IS A DESIGNER AND ILLUSTRATOR WHO LIVES SOMETIMES IN AUSTIN, TEXAS, SOMETIMES IN ZÜRICH, SWITZERLAND, AND ALWAYS WITH HER PARTNER, COLIN, AND THEIR DOG, LUNA. TO SEE MORE OF HER ART, GO TO JENNALUECKE.COM OR @JENNALUECKE ON INSTAGRAM.

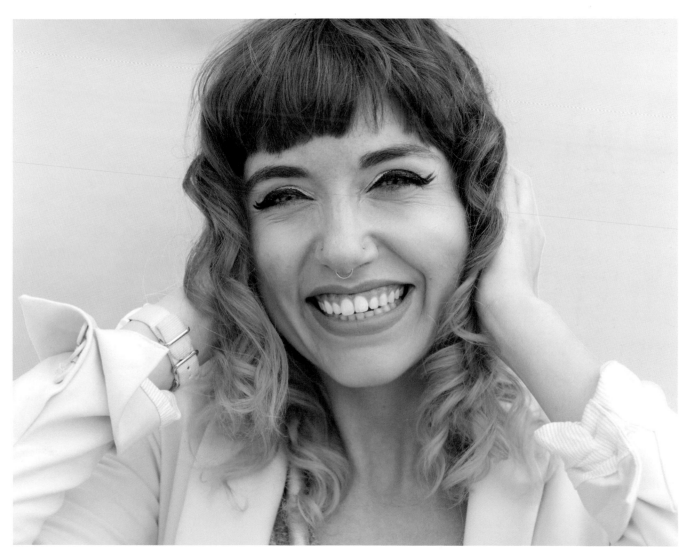

THE BREAKUP HAIR HANDBOOK

Andrews McMeel Publishing
a division of Andrews McMeel Universal
1130 Walnut Street, Kansas City, Missouri 64106

www.andrewsmcmeel.com

20 21 22 23 24 SHO 10 9 8 7 6 5 4 3 2 1

ISBN: 978-1-5248-5888-9

Library of Congress Control Number: 2020937574

Editor: Allison Adler
Art Director: Holly Swayne
Production Editor: Julie Railsback
Production Manager: Carol Coe

ATTENTION: SCHOOLS AND BUSINESSES
Andrews McMeel books are available at quantity discounts with bulk purchase
for educational, business, or sales promotional use. For information,
please e-mail the Andrews McMeel Publishing Special Sales Department:
specialsales@amuniversal.com.